I0415323

The Ultimate Alzheimer's Prevention Cookbook

Complete Guide for Alzheimer's Caregivers

BY: Allie Allen

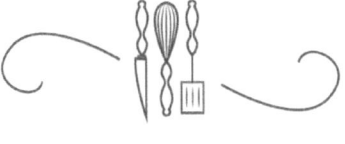

COOK & ENJOY

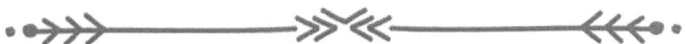

Copyright Notes

This book is written as an informational tool. While the author has taken every precaution to ensure the accuracy of the information provided therein, the reader is warned that they assume all risk when following the content. The author will not be held responsible for any damages that may occur as a result of the readers' actions.

The author does not give permission to reproduce this book in any form, including but not limited to: print, social media posts, electronic copies or photocopies, unless permission is expressly given in writing.

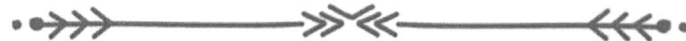

My Gift to You for Buying My Book!

I would like to extend an exclusive offer to receive free and discounted eBooks every day! This special gift is my way of saying thanks. If you fill in the subscription box below you will begin to receive special offers directly to your email.

Not only that! You will also receive notifications letting you know when an offer will expire. You will never miss a chance to get a free book! Who wouldn't want that?

Fill in the subscriber information below and get started today!

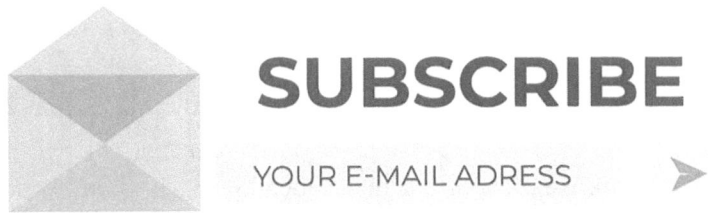

https://allie-allen.getresponsepages.com/

Table of Contents

Alzheimer's Prevention Recipes.................................... 6

1) Stuffed Zucchini with Beef and Grapes 7

2) Fish Filets with its little Vegetables............................... 10

3) Spanish Style Fish Cutlets 12

4) Pork Fillet with Leeks and Caramelized Apple.............. 14

5) Celery and Apple Soup.. 17

6) Smoked Trout and Apple Salad...................................... 19

7) Tomato and Pepper Ice.. 21

8) My 'Ota'ika.. 24

9) Haddock and Pear with a Ginger Vinaigrette 26

10) Monkfish Tartar with Avocado, Strawberries and Watermelon.. 28

11) Zucchini, Eggplant and Beans Salad............................ 31

12) Minted Pesto Lamb Salad 33

13) Smoked Chicken Salad.................................. 35

14) Mediterranean Peppers Salad 37

15) Avocado Caesar Salad................................. 39

16) Marinated Sardines with Tomatoes and Raisins............ 42

17) Crispy Papillote of Whiting 44

18) Honey Salmon Steaks with a Sesame Rocket Salad 46

19) Grilled Chicken with Endives, Cashew Salad.............. 48

20) Crab Salad with Tomato Dressing 51

21) Lentils and Bulgur Rosti with Yogurt Dressing 54

22) Chicken Casserole..................................... 58

23) Lamb with Black Olives 60

24) Chicken Mediterranean Casserole 62

25) Sautéed Calamari 65

About the Author.................................. 67

Author's Afterthoughts.. 69

Alzheimer's Prevention

Recipes

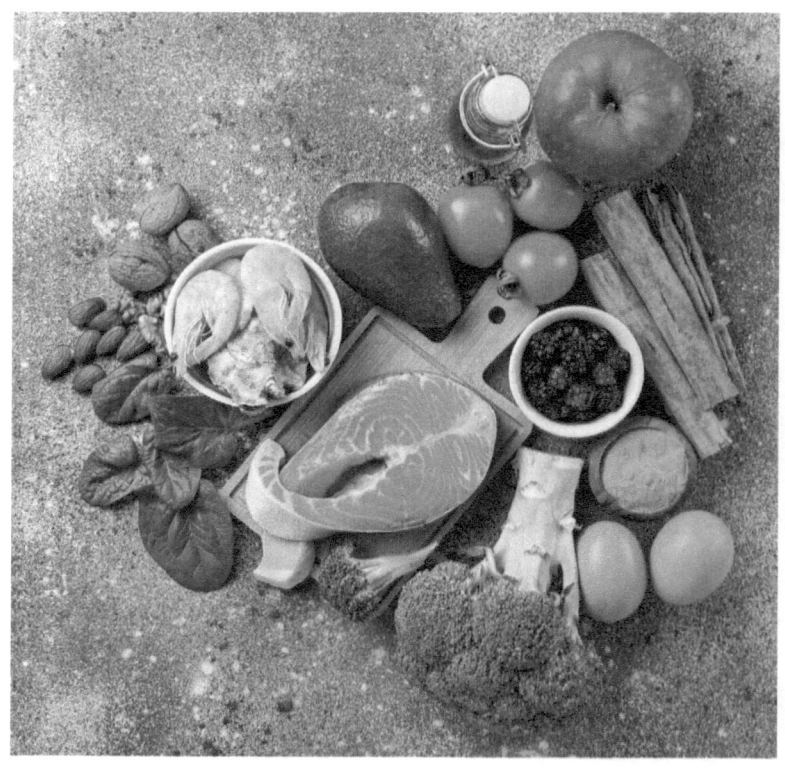

ssssssssssssssssssssssssssssssssssssssssssssssssssssss

1) Stuffed Zucchini with Beef and Grapes

Meat is an essential part of our life diet. Do not stop eating meat. Eat moderately and choose lean pieces, beef is very nutritious food. It contains high quality proteins; it is an excellent source of 12 vitamins and minerals as well, including iron and zinc.

Yield: 4

Cooking Time: 1 hour 10 minutes

List of Ingredients:

- 7/8 lb. of minced beef
- 8 round zucchini
- 1 onion, chopped
- 2 garlic cloves, chopped
- 4 oz. of grapes, cut in halves
- 2 tbsp. of olive oil
- 7/8 cup of red wine
- 1 bunch of parsley, chopped
- 2 tomatoes, cut in pieces
- Salt and pepper

sssssssssssssssssssssssssssssssssssssssssssssssss

Instructions:

Preheat the oven at 350 F.

Warm up the olive oil in a frying pan.

Add and sweet the onion and garlic until tender.

Add the beef and cook for 3 to 4 minutes.

Meanwhile, cut the top of the zucchini and empty the inside without cutting through.

Add the inside of the zucchini in the frying pan.

Add the grapes, tomatoes and red wine as well.

Cook for 5 minutes gently and season.

Fill the beef mixture in each round zucchini.

Put the top as a lid and place all in an oven dish.

Cook in the oven for 45 minutes.

Serve two per person and enjoy.

2) Fish Filets with its little Vegetables

Full flavor is on; your taste bud will be delighted by this smooth taste. Don't hesitate to add other vegetable if you want and if you do, please, adjust the quantity of liquid too. Serve it with a mixed salad or even a nice homemade mash potato.

Yield: 4

Cooking Time: 40 minutes

List of Ingredients:

- 4 filets of white fish, like cod, etc.
- 1 leeks, finely slice
- 2 carrots, finely slice
- 1 shallot, chopped
- 1 tbsp. of olive oil
- 1 glass of white wine
- 3 tbsp. of single cream
- 1 tsp. of thyme
- Salt and pepper

ss

Instructions:

Preheat the oven at 350 F.

Heat the olive oil in a frying pan.

Add and sweat the shallot until tender.

Add the leeks and carrots and cook for 5 minutes at low heat.

Stirring occasionally pour the white wine and reduce for another 5 minutes.

Add the cream and season.

Place the fish filets first in four small individual oven dishes.

Cover with vegetable mixture.

Sprinkle on the top with thyme.

Cook in the oven for 15 to 20 minutes.

Serve hot and enjoy.

3) Spanish Style Fish Cutlets

The mackerel is one of the fish so rich in omega 3. It also provides useful amounts of vitamins B and D, as well as several minerals. Like the sardines, it is recommended to pregnant women. Available all year round and it is an easy fish to create variety of recipes.

Yield: 4

Cooking Time: 45 minutes

List of Ingredients:

- 4 jewfish cutlets
- 4 tbsp. of olive oil
- 1 tbsp. of parsley, chopped
- 3 garlic cloves, crushed
- 1 oz. of almonds, slivered
- 1 tbsp. of green onions, chopped
- ½ tsp. of paprika
- ½ tsp. of lemon rind, grated
- 6 plum tomatoes
- Salt and pepper

sss

Instructions:

Preheat the oven at 350F.

Brush both sides of the fish with the olive oil.

Place the fish cutlets on an oven tray.

Mix the rest of the olive oil with the garlic in a bowl.

Add the parsley, paprika, almonds, lemon rind, and green onions.

Cover the top of each cutlet with the mixture on the oven dish.

Add the plum tomatoes on the side of the fish.

Place the dish in the oven and cook for 20 minutes.

Make sure the fish is cooked or leave it a little longer.

Serve immediately and enjoy.

4) Pork Fillet with Leeks and Caramelized Apple

The leek is one of the few vegetables that can be found all year round thanks to its different varieties and also because it is resistant to cold winter. It is in this season when the leek is the most useful because it is very rich in vitamins and minerals.

Yield: 4

Cooking Time: 40 minutes

List of Ingredients:

- 4 pork fillet or tenderloin
- 4 apple, cut in quarters
- 2 leeks, shredded
- 1 garlic clove, finely chopped
- ¾ cup of chicken stock
- 4 tbsp. of red wine
- 2 knob of butter
- 2 tbsp. of olive oil
- 1 tbsp. of honey

- Salt and pepper

ssssssssssssssssssssssssssssssssssssssssssssssssssss

Instructions:

Warm up the butter in a large frying pan.

Add the honey and mix well and add after the apple.

Cook gently at low heat until the apples are caramelizing.

Turn the apple often.

Leave on the side to cool down.

Heat the olive oil in another frying pan.

Add the garlic and cook for 2 minutes.

Add the pork fillet and cook on both sides thoroughly.

Remove the pork and keep warm.

Deglaze with the red wine.

Add the chicken stock and leave on a medium heat.

Add the leek and cook until the liquid is reduced and is thicker.

Put the leeks on the plate first and the pork after.

Add some caramelized apples on the top and enjoy.

5) Celery and Apple Soup

This interesting combination of flavors produces a tasty soup. Remember to serve it with some nice country bread - it would be perfect. The best is to use cooking apples but you can use the other variety too. Keep some bits of apple and celery to garnish the soup in the end.

Yield: 4

Cooking Time: 55 minutes

List of Ingredients:

- 2 tbsp. of olive oil
- 1 large onion, finely chopped
- 3 cooking apple, sliced
- 2 pints of vegetable stock
- 1 bay leaf
- 3 sticks of celery, finely chopped
- Salt and pepper

sssssssssssssssssssssssssssssssssssssssssssssssssssss

Instructions:

Warm up the olive oil in a large pan.

Add and sweat the onion until they turn soft but not brown.

Add the apple and cook for 3 minutes until the apple starts to soften.

Add the vegetable stock and the bay leaf.

Add the celery and season. Bring to the boiling stage.

Cover and simmer for 30 minutes on medium heat.

Blend the soup until smooth.

Return to the heat and bring back to the boil.

Serve hot and enjoy it.

6) Smoked Trout and Apple Salad

We never eat enough of fruits during the day so why not to add them to our lunch or dinner. Here you have a perfect example of a salad and, to be honest, if you add some other fruit too, like pineapple, orange, grapefruit, they will all go perfectly with this salad. Enjoy it!

Yield: 4

Cooking Time: 20 minutes

List of Ingredients:

- 3 apples
- 6 oz. smoked trout
- ½ cup of natural yogurts
- 1 oak leaf salad or any other of your choice
- 3 tbsp. of lemon juice
- 1 tbsp. of chives
- 2 tbsp. of parmesan
- Salt and pepper

SSS

Instructions:

Cut the apple into quarters and remove the cores.

Leave the skin of the apples on.

Slice the apple into a bowl and mix with two tbsp. of lemon juice.

Wash, drain and break the oak leaf salad into a large bowl.

Skin the trout and take off any bones you notice.

Flake the trout into large pieces. Leave on the side.

Whisk the yogurt with one tbsp. of lemon juice in a small bowl.

Add the parmesan and season.

Add the apple and the trout with the oak leaf salad.

Drizzle some of the yogurt dressing with it and mix well.

Keep some dressing on the side and serve.

7) Tomato and Pepper Ice

Similar to frozen Gazpacho, this original appetizer is ideal for serving in warm summer days. It could be used in smaller quantities as well, as a palate freshener courses to replace conventional sorbet. Be careful not to allow the tomato ice to freeze into a solid block.

Yield: 4

Cooking Time: 15 minutes + freezing time

List of Ingredients:

- 6 ice cubes
- ½ cup of tomato juice
- 1 lemon, juice
- 1 tsp. of Worcester sauce
- 1 green pepper, seeded and finely chopped
- 1 red pepper, seeded and finely chopped
- 4 tomatoes
- Salt and pepper

ssssssssssssssssssssssssssssssssssssssssssssssssssssssss

Instructions:

Cut the top of the tomatoes and keep the hat on the side.

Scoop out the inside and keep on the side.

Put the inside of the tomatoes into a blender.

Add the tomato juice, lemon juice and Worcester sauce.

Break the ice cubes into small pieces and add to the blender.

Blend until it becomes a smooth slush.

Pour the mixture into an ice tray and freeze for ½ hour or until it just begins to freeze.

Pour the freezing mixture into a bowl and mash until the crystals are well broken up.

Mix it with the green and red peppers and return it into the ice tray.

Re-freeze further for another one and half an hour.

Stir occasionally to prevent the mixture from solidifying completely.

To serve it allows 5 minutes for the mixture to defrost then mash it with a back of a fork.

Fill the mixture inside the chilled tomato shells.

Serve immediately.

8) My 'Ota'ika

The fish is raw so try to choose a variety of fish which has a firm flesh such as tuna, sea bream, etc. If you place the fish in the freezer for few minutes before cutting you will find the process to be very easy. Serve with a green salad on the side. This recipe is originated from Tahiti.

Yield: 6

Cooking Time: 25 minutes

List of Ingredients:

- 1.5 lb. of fresh fish
- 6 limes, juice
- 3 tbsp. of olive oil
- 2 tomatoes
- 2 carrots
- ½ cucumber
- 1 onion
- 6 tbsp. of coconut, grated
- Salt and pepper

sssssssssssssssssssssssssssssssssssssssssssssssssssssss

Instructions:

Cut the fish into thin strips and place them in a large bowl.

Fill the bowl with salty water and leave in the fridge.

Peel and cut the onion into very small dices and do the same with the tomatoes.

Cut the cucumber into very small dices too.

Grate the carrots and leave on the side.

Drain the fish and rinse it with clear water.

Squeeze the lime into the fish and add the olive oil.

Mix well and season.

Add the cucumber, tomatoes, onion, and carrots.

Add the grated coconut and mix well.

Leave the fish mixture in the fridge before serving.

9) Haddock and Pear with a Ginger Vinaigrette

Fish combines with fruits very easily as an appetizer or main course - you will enjoy the combination. Make sure it's very fresh; put it in the fridge for 30 minutes before serving. You can add some green like rocket salad for example or another one.

Yield: 4

Cooking Time: 25 minutes

List of Ingredients:

- 7/8 lb. haddock
- 2 pears Williams
- ½ bunch of chives, chopped
- 1 tsp. of ginger, grated
- 1 lime, juice
- 1 tbsp. of honey
- 6 tbsp. of olive oil
- Salt and pepper

sss

Instructions:

Peel the pears, cut into quarters, remove the heart and seeds and then cut into small cubes.

Cut the haddock into small cubes, the same way as the pears.

Place the haddock, the pears and the chives in a bowl and mix well.

Pour the lime juice and the olive oil in another bowl.

Add the ginger and the honey.

Mix well all the ingredients and season.

Place two tbsp. of the mix haddock and pear in the center of the plate.

Drizzle some of the ginger vinaigrette.

Serve and enjoy it.

10) Monkfish Tartar with Avocado, Strawberries and Watermelon

You will get an explosion of flavor with this recipe. The monkfish is raw but you can cook it if you prefer but remember to place the fish cold with the other ingredients. You can mix the fish with some olive oil as well before you do the tartar.

Yield: 4

Cooking Time: 25 minutes

List of Ingredients:

- ½ lb. of monkfish filets
- 8 strawberries
- ¼ watermelon
- 2 avocado
- 1 lemon
- 1 red onion
- 4 tbsp. of olive oil
- 1 tbsp. of vinegar
- 1 tsp. of honey
- Salt and pepper

sssssssssssssssssssssssssssssssssssssssssssssssssssss

Instructions:

Cut the monkfish into very small cubes. Season.

Cut the strawberries into small pieces.

Cut the watermelon into small cubes.

Peel and cut the red onion very thinly.

Cut the avocado into small pieces and mix with the lemon juice.

Climb the tartar with a kitchen metal circle.

First layer the avocado and layer the fish after.

Finish with mix strawberries and watermelon.

Mix the olive oil and vinegar in a bowl.

Add the honey and red onion. Season and mix well.

Pour the dressing on the plate all around the tartar.

Serve chill and enjoy.

11) Zucchini, Eggplant and Beans Salad

Classic from the Mediterranean cuisine the eggplant is very low in calories and is healthy as it reduces the risk of certain diseases. This salad can be enjoyed hot or cold and if you decide to taste it hot so add the beans with the garlic and cumin seeds, grill the tomatoes too.

Yield: 4

Cooking Time: 40 minutes

List of Ingredients:

- 3 small zucchini
- 2 medium eggplant
- 8 cherry tomatoes, cut in halves
- 1 tbsp. of cumin seeds
- ½ cup of olive oil
- 1/3 cup of lemon juice
- 2 garlic cloves
- ¾ lb. of cannellini beans, rinsed and drained
- ½ cup of fresh coriander leaves

- Salt and pepper

ssssssssssssssssssssssssssssssssssssssssssssssssssssssss

Instructions:

Cut the zucchini lengthwise and slice the eggplant.

Brush all the pieces of zucchini and eggplant with olive oil.

Grill all until browned on both sides and tender.

Warm up the rest of the olive oil in a frying pan.

Add the garlic and cumin seeds and cook for 2 to 3 minutes.

Combine the zucchini and eggplant in a large serving bowl.

Add the cherry tomatoes and the beans.

Pour the garlic and cumin seeds to it.

Add the coriander and lemon juice. Season well.

Mix gently everything and serve.

12) Minted Pesto Lamb Salad

Make sure you made enough minted pesto dressing since people always ask for more. The lamb must be pink and cold but you can always have it warm too. The same for the peppers. Cook longer if you prefer tender and not crunchy.

Yield: 4

Cooking Time: 20 minutes

List of Ingredients:

- 1.5 lb. lamb, cooked and sliced
- 1 onion, sliced
- 2 garlic cloves, crushed
- 1 salad of your choice
- 1 red pepper, cut into strips
- 1 yellow pepper, cut into strips
- 2 tbsp. of pine nuts
- 2 oz. of fresh basil
- 1 oz. of fresh mints
- ½ cup of olive oil
- Salt and pepper

sss

Instructions:

Prepare the salad of your choice in a large bowl.

Add red and yellow peppers.

Add the onion and mix well.

Put the pine nuts, basil, and mints in a blender. Season.

Start blending and add the olive oil little by little until you get a smooth paste.

Put four portions of salad on four plates.

Add the slice of lamb on the top.

Drizzle some of the minted pesto on each plate.

Serve and enjoy.

13) Smoked Chicken Salad

Smoked chicken has already been cooked during the curing process, making this a simple salad to throw together at short notice. You can keep the smoked chicken in the freezer. Try to use a natural local honey without any other things added to it.

Yield: 4

Cooking Time: 15 minutes

List of Ingredients:

- ½ lb. of baby spinach leaves
- 1 oak leaf salad
- 7/8 lb. of smoked chicken breast, sliced
- 1 yellow pepper
- 1 red onion
- 1 cup of basil leaves
- ¼ cup of lime juice
- 1 tbsp. of honey
- 1 small red chili, seeded, chopped finely
- 2 tbsp. of olive oil

- Salt and pepper

sssssssssssssssssssssssssssssssssssssssssssssssssssssss

Instructions:

Wash and drain the oak leaf and baby spinach.

Mix together and put the salad in a large serving bowl.

Slice the yellow pepper and red onion thinly.

Add to the salad with the basil and mix together.

Add the smoked chicken to it.

Mix the olive oil and lime juice in a small bowl.

Add the honey and red chili. Season.

Whisk thoroughly the mixture.

Pour the dressing to the salad and mix well everything.

Serve and enjoy it.

14) Mediterranean Peppers Salad

A full flavor recipe with so many different colors - this salad really gives you the warmth of the Mediterranean coast. You can add some cubes of cheese or some pieces of fish too, like tuna or salmon - the choice is yours. Eat as much as you want; it is very healthy for you.

Yield: 4

Cooking Time: 45 minutes

List of Ingredients:

- 1 onion, thinly chopped
- 2 red peppers, cut into strips
- 2 yellow peppers, cut into strips
- 2 green peppers, cut into strips
- 1 zucchini, sliced
- 2 garlic cloves, chopped
- 1 oz. of stoned black olive, halves
- 10 cherry tomatoes, cut in halves
- 3 tbsp. of olive oil

- 1 tbsp. of balsamic vinegar
- 1 tbsp. of basil
- Salt and pepper

sssssssssssssssssssssssssssssssssssssssssssssssssssssssss

Instructions:

Warm up the olive oil in a large frying pan.

Add and sweat the onion and garlic until tender.

Add the green, red, and yellow peppers with the zucchini.

Cook for 20 minutes on low heat and stir occasionally.

Add the black olives and tomato cherry.

Add the basil and vinegar. Season. Mix well.

Cook further for another5 minutes and stir occasionally.

Serve on the top or on the side of a mixed salad.

15) Avocado Caesar Salad

This is a different way of doing the classic Caesar salad recipe. Remember, instead of avocado you can always add some grilled chicken too or even both. You can do the croutons a day before if you have time barriers, but for myself, I prefer doing on the same day - they are crustier and not hard.

Yield: 4

Cooking Time: 30 minutes

List of Ingredients:

- 1 romaine lettuce
- 2 avocado, sliced
- 1 red onion, sliced
- 3 garlic clove, thinly chopped
- 2 tbsp. of parsley, finely chopped
- 4 slices of bread, cut into cubes
- 2 eggs York
- 8 tbsp. of olive oil
- 1 tbsp. of mustard
- 8 anchovies
- 4 tbsp. of parmesan, grated
- Salt and pepper

SSSSSSSSSSSSSSSSSSSSSSSSSSSSSSSSSSSSSSSSSSSSSSSSSSSS

Instructions:

Warm up two tbsp. of olive oil in a frying pan.

Add two garlic cloves and the parsley.

Cook for 2 to 3 minutes and after add the small bread cubes.

Cook until the bread is golden brown and leave on the side.

Put the rest of the garlic, anchovies, and mustard in a blender.

Add the eggs yolk and start mixing.

Gradually add the rest of the olive oil until you get a smooth mixture. Season.

Add more olive oil if you don't like the level of thickness.

Mix the dressing with the romaine lettuce in a large bowl.

Add the red onion and croutons "bread".

Add the avocado and mix very gently.

Sprinkle the parmesan and serve.

16) Marinated Sardines with Tomatoes and Raisins

Serve the tasteful appetizer with some crusty bread, so perfect. You can always add some cucumber too. You can as well replace the raisins with fresh grapes if the season allows it, will be even better. Remember fresh food is always the best.

Yield: 4

Cooking Time: 25 minutes

List of Ingredients:

- 16 small filets of fresh sardines
- ½ cup of dry raisins
- 6 pitted black olives, cut into halves
- 2 tomato
- 1 lemon, juice
- 6 tbsp. of olive oil
- 4 sprigs of fresh thyme
- 3 tbsp. of white wine
- Salt and pepper

ss

Instructions:

Cut the sardines filets into small pieces.

Place the cut sardines in a flat dish.

Mix the olive oil and the lemon juice in a bowl.

Add the raisins and the thyme. Season.

Put the tomatoes for few minutes in boiling water.

Drain and peel them. Crush the tomatoes and add to the marinade.

Add the black olive and white wine.

Mix well and pour on the top of the sardines.

Place and leave in the fridge for at least one hour.

Serve equal portions for everyone and enjoy.

17) Crispy Papillote of Whiting

Instead of using the traditional cooking paper for the papillote use some filo pastry; a very interesting change. Cooking in papillote is always very easy and most of the results are very good. Serve it with a nice salad and some quarters of lemon for garnish.

Yield: 4

Cooking Time: 25 minutes

List of Ingredients:

- 4 whiting filets
- 3 carrots, finely slice
- 1 leek, finely slice
- 5 garlic cloves, thinly chopped
- 4 sheets of filo pastry
- 4 tbsp. of white wine
- 1 sprigs of thyme
- Salt and pepper

ssssssssssssssssssssssssssssssssssssssssssssssssssssss

Instructions:

Preheat the oven at 350 F.

Season the fish filets on each side.

Spread the filo pastry sheets on a work surface.

Place the whiting filet on each of the pastry sheets.

Add equally the leeks, carrots and garlic.

Pour the white wine and put some thyme on the fish.

Gently fold the edges of the filo pastry and tie the end with either some kitchen string or wooden pick.

Brush the papillotes with olive oil.

Cook in the oven for 10 minutes.

Serve hot and enjoy it.

18) Honey Salmon Steaks with a Sesame Rocket Salad

This is a light recipe but you have to be very quick in it. By mixing honey and olive oil together the salmon will take the flavor of the honey - you will be very surprised with the result. You can do the same with herbs such as thyme and coriander as well.

Yield: 4

Cooking Time: 20 minutes

List of Ingredients:

- 4 salmon steak
- 2 tbsp. of lemon juice
- 3 tbsp. of olive oil
- 3 tbsp. of honey
- 2 tbsp. of sesame seeds
- 1 bag of rocket salad
- 1 lemon, cut into quarters for garnish

sssssssssssssssssssssssssssssssssssssssssssssssssssss

Instructions:

Warm up the olive oil in a frying pan.

Add the honey and mix well.

When the oil is very hot, place the salmon steaks with the skin first to cook.

Cook for 3 to 4 minutes on each side depending on the thickness of your salmon.

Meanwhile, put your rocket salad in a large serving bowl.

As soon as your salmon steaks are done remove them from the heat and keep warm.

Add the sesame seeds and cook for 1 to 2 minutes in the same frying pan.

Deglaze quickly with the lemon juice.

And pour the dressing onto the rocket salad.

Mix well and season.

Serve the salmon either on the top of the rocket salad or on the side.

19) Grilled Chicken with Endives, Cashew Salad

The endive is a particularly low-calorie leafy vegetable. It is a good source of minerals and it is particularly useful for pregnant women or women who wish to conceive. You can either eat it raw or cooked, as a salad or in "gratin" bake.

Yield: 4

Cooking Time: 35 minutes

List of Ingredients:

- 2 endives, shredded
- ½ cos lettuce, shredded
- 4 chicken breasts
- 2 tbsp. of olive oil
- 1 red onion, sliced
- 1 cup of unsalted cashew
- 1 cup of dry raisins
- 1 cup of yogurt
- 2 garlic cloves, finely chopped
- ¼ cup of lemon juice
- ¼ cup of coriander, chopped
- Salt and pepper

sssssssssssssssssssssssssssssssssssssssssssssssssssss

Instructions:

Flat the chicken breasts with a kitchen hammer or with your roll pin.

Brush the chicken with the olive oil.

Cook the flat chicken under the grill until it is done.

Combine the yogurt with the garlic, lemon juice, and coriander in a bowl.

Mix well and leave on the side.

Combine the endives with the cos lettuce in a large serving bowl.

Add the red onion, cashew and raisins. Mix well everything.

Toss gently to combine the yogurt dressing with the salad.

Slice the grill chicken and place it on the top of the salad.

Serve and enjoy it.

20) Crab Salad with Tomato Dressing

This chubby bulb vegetable is full of water and valuable minerals including potassium and magnesium. The calcium is also very high. It displays a level of iron well above the average and is a champion on vitamin C, E and B9. So, don't wait and eat some fennel, get used to it and enjoy.

Yield: 4

Cooking Time: 35 minutes

List of Ingredients:

- 9 oz. of fresh crab or canned crab meat
- 1 large bulb fennel, thinly sliced
- 3 oz. of mixed salad leaves
- 1 tbsp. of chives
- 1 tbsp. of paprika
- 2 large tomatoes
- 2 tbsp. of tomato juice
- 5 tbsp. of olive oil
- 1 tsp. of tarragon
- ½ cucumber, cut into very small diced
- Dash of Worcester sauce
- 1 tbsp. of balsamic vinegar

SSSSSSSSSSSSSSSSSSSSSSSSSSSSSSSSSSSSSSSSSSSSSSSSSSS

Instructions:

Place the tomatoes in a bowl and cover with hot water.

Leave for 30 seconds, then skin, deseed and cut the tomatoes into small dices.

While cutting the tomatoes keep the juice from them and add to the dressing after.

Whisk the olive oil with the balsamic vinegar in a small bowl.

Add the tarragon, Worcester sauce, and the tomato juice. Season.

Mix the crab meat with the fennel in a large bowl.

Add the dice tomatoes and cucumber. Mix well.

Pour the tomato dressing over the crab salad and mix.

Serve with a mixed salad leaves on the side.

21) Lentils and Bulgur Rosti with Yogurt Dressing

Rosti can be made with all sort of different ingredients and not always potatoes. Make it as thick as you want, obviously the thicker you do the longer it need to cook on each side. If you cannot find some bulgur use another cereal.

Yield: 4

Cooking Time: 1 hour 10 minutes

List of Ingredients:

- 1/3 lb. of lentils
- ¼ lb. of bulgur
- 5 tbsp. of olive oil
- 1 onion, finely chopped
- 3 tsp. of cumin
- 2 tsp. of powder coriander
- 3 tbsp. of fresh mints
- 4 eggs, beaten
- ½ cup of flour
- 1 small cucumber, cut into very small cubes
- ½ cup of yogurt
- 1 garlic clove, thinly chopped
- Salt and pepper

sssssssssssssssssssssssssssssssssssssssssssssssss

Instructions:

Heat a pan with boiling water.

Add the lentils and cook for 30 minutes until tender.

Stop the cooking and make sure there is just enough water covering the lentils.

Add the bulgur on it and leave on the side for at least 1 hour and 30 minutes.

Meanwhile, mix the yogurt with the garlic and cucumber in a bowl.

After one and half hour add the onion, cumin, mints, coriander, eggs, and flour in the pan.

Mix everything until you get a compact composition.

Warm up the olive oil in a large frying pan on medium heat.

Place some of the compact mixture forming a rosti with a large spoon.

Cook both sides until golden brown for around 2 minutes on each side.

Repeat until you use all of the compact mixture.

Serve with the yogurt dressing on the side.

22) Chicken Casserole

The chicken can be prepared and enjoyed in thousands of different ways. But sometimes it is industrially deformed to the point that only the word "chicken" on the packaging enables us to know what it is … it's a shame! So give yourself the pleasure of a real chicken and enjoy without excess.

Yield: 4

Cooking Time: 1 hour 10 minutes

List of Ingredients:

- 1 whole chicken, cut into 8 pieces
- 2 tbsp. of olive oil
- 1 onion, chopped
- 2 garlic cloves, crushed
- 1 green and red peppers, cut in strips
- 1 large canned of chopped tomatoes
- 4 large potatoes, cut into four pieces each of them
- ½ cup of white wine
- 6 oz. of black olives, stoned
- 1 tbsp. of thyme

- 1 bay leaf
- Salt and pepper

sssssssssssssssssssssssssssssssssssssssssssssssssss

Instructions:

Warm up olive oil in a large sauce pan.

Place the chicken pieces and fry until golden brown on all sides.

Remove and keep on the side.

Add and sweat the onion and garlic until tender.

Add the green and red peppers and tomatoes.

Add the chicken pieces back into the pan.

Pour the white wine and add the thyme and bay leaf.

Add black olives and potatoes. Season.

Bring to the boil and reduce to low heat.

Cook and simmer for 45 minutes. Stir occasionally.

Serve immediately and enjoy it.

23) Lamb with Black Olives

A very tasty and slightly hot lamb recipe which I am sure you will enjoy. Although high in saturated fat, lamb is a good source of protein but also of zinc, a mineral that affects many fundamental processes going on in our body, without doubt the most important immune function. You can serve this dish with any vegetable and potatoes of your choice.

Yield: 4

Cooking Time: 35 minutes

List of Ingredients:

- 12 oz. boned leg of lamb, cut into cube
- 4 tbsp. of olive oil
- 2 garlic cloves, crushed and chopped
- 1 onion, chopped
- 1 small red chili, deseeded and chopped finely
- ½ cup of white wine
- 6 oz. of stoned black olives
- 1 sprigs of parsley, chopped
- 1 tbsp. of rosemary
- Salt and pepper

SSS

Instructions:

Warm up the olive oil in a large frying pan

Add and sweat the onion, garlic and red chili until tender.

Add the lamb and brown from all sides being careful not to burn it.

Deglaze with the white wine for 2 to 3 minutes.

Add the black olive and reduce the heat to medium.

Add the rosemary and season.

Cook and simmer for 20 minutes.

Stir occasionally during the last 5 minutes, add half of the parsley.

Transfer the lamb into a serving dish.

Sprinkle the rest of the parsley and enjoy it.

24) Chicken Mediterranean Casserole

Use as much different vegetable as you wish with this recipe but don't add any potato. You can serve it with rice but really much better on its own. This recipe can be done with pork as well just replace the chicken and don't change anything else.

Yield: 4

Cooking Time: 1 hour 20 minutes

List of Ingredients:

- 1 whole chicken cut into 8 pieces
- 1 onion, chopped
- 2 garlic cloves, crushed
- 1 zucchini, sliced
- 1 yellow pepper, cut into strips
- 1 red pepper, cut into strips
- 6 oz. of bottom mushrooms, sliced
- 6 tomatoes, sliced
- 1 Tbsp. of thyme
- 1 bay leaf

- 4 oz. of green olives, stoned
- ½ cut of red wine
- ½ cut of chicken stock
- 2 tbsp. of olive oil
- Salt and pepper

sssssssssssssssssssssssssssssssssssssssssssssssssss

Instructions:

Preheat the oven at 350 F.

Warm up the olive oil in a large sauce pan.

Fry the chicken pieces on each side until they have a nice golden brown color.

Remove the chicken and place in the oven dish.

Add and sweat the onion and garlic until tender.

Put the onion and garlic into the oven dish.

Add the red and yellow peppers, and zucchini.

Add the mushrooms, tomatoes, and the green olives.

Add the thyme and bay leaf. Season.

Pour the red wine and the chicken stock.

Cook and simmer in the oven for 45 minutes.

Remove from the oven and make sure the chicken is thoroughly cooked.

Serve immediately.

25) Sautéed Calamari

The calamari can be cooked in many different recipes and there are many ways to enjoy it - fried, stuffed, grilled, etc. It will change your everyday recipes by adding something different to your accepted list of ingredients. You can either buy calamari fresh or frozen. It is best to serve the dish with rice or a mix salad.

Yield: 4

Cooking Time: 20 minutes

List of Ingredients:

- 18 oz. of calamari ring
- 3 tbsp. of olive oil
- 1 onion, chopped
- 2 garlic cloves, crushed
- 1 tbsp. of basil
- 1 tbsp. of madras mild curry
- 1 tbsp. of parsley
- 2 tbsp. of honey
- 2 canned of chopped tomatoes with juice
- Salt and pepper

ss

Instructions:

Warm up the olive oil in a large frying pan.

Add and sweat the onion and garlic until tender.

Add the madras, basil, and honey. Mix well.

Add the tomatoes and season.

Add the calamari ring and mix well everything.

Cook gently for 5 minutes and stir occasionally.

Add the parsley in the end and serve.

About the Author

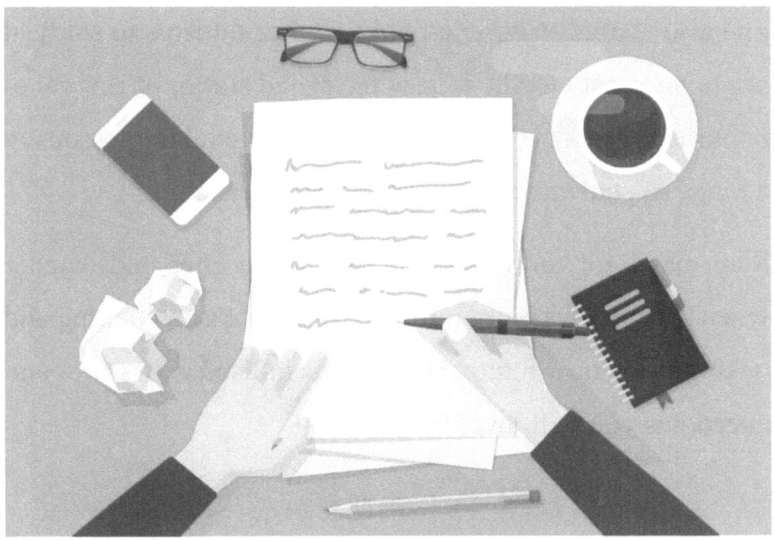

Allie Allen developed her passion for the culinary arts at the tender age of five when she would help her mother cook for their large family of 8. Even back then, her family knew this would be more than a hobby for the young Allie and when she graduated from high school, she applied to cooking school in London. It had always been a dream of the young chef to study with some of Europe's best and she made it happen by attending the Chef Academy of London.

After graduation, Allie decided to bring her skills back to North America and open up her own restaurant. After 10 successful years as head chef and owner, she decided to sell her business and pursue other career avenues. This monumental decision led Allie to her true calling, teaching. She also started to write e-books for her students to study at home for practice. She is now the proud author of several e-books and gives private and semi-private cooking lessons to a range of students at all levels of experience.

Stay tuned for more from this dynamic chef and teacher when she releases more informative e-books on cooking and baking in the near future. Her work is infused with stores and anecdotes you will love!

Author's Afterthoughts

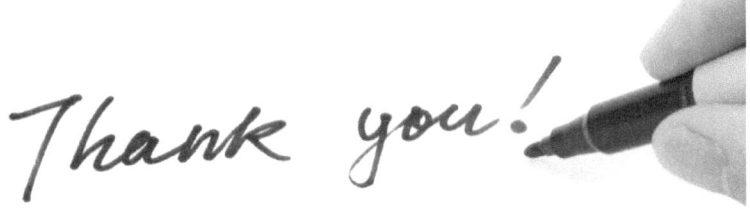

I can't tell you how grateful I am that you decided to read my book. My most heartfelt thanks that you took time out of your life to choose my work and I hope you find benefit within these pages.

There are so many books available today that offer similar content so that makes it even more humbling that you decided to buying mine.

Tell me what you thought! I am eager to hear your opinion and ideas on what you read as are others who are looking for a good book to buy. Leave a review on Amazon.com so others can benefit from your wisdom!

With much thanks,

Allie Allen

www.ingramcontent.com/pod-product-compliance
Lightning Source LLC
Chambersburg PA
CBHW021249280526
45784CB00005B/2297